"Absolutely Brilliant!" - Nick V

I'm Daisy the Safety Chihuahua

Safety Tips for Children

By Diana Trepkov
Forensic Artist

Chihuahua Teaches Important Safety Rules in Delightful Picture Book

Author pens adorable safety children's book that appeals to the child in everyone

When a child goes missing, it is every parent's worst nightmare. Nothing is more important to a mother and father than their children's safety and welfare. While they can't protect them 24/7, the least they can do is to educate them so they can protect themselves when there is a potential threat. Author Diana Trepkov offers safety tips for children as she shares *I'm Daisy, the Safety Chihuahua.*

This picture book introduces Daisy, who might look like an ordinary Chihuahua but is actually a safety Chihuahua. She teaches kids how to stay safe by sharing important safety rules that are smart and easy to remember. She also shares tips like how getting a good night's sleep can help one make wise decisions or how bullying is a bad thing. Some of the essential things that children should remember are to never talk to strangers and to always listen to their intuition and gut feelings.

The author shares, "It is a wish I have deep within myself, and that is to protect as many children as possible, to help ease the pain that I have witnessed in so many families' eyes of missing loved ones. This is written from my heart and through my eyes, the eyes of a forensic artist."

With *I'm Daisy, the Safety* Chihuahua, colorful photographs, detailed illustrations, important safety tips, and fun activities are all wrapped up in one small fun package. Children of all ages will treasure this book of inspiration, safety rules, and assurance through their journey in life. This adorable safety children's book will also appeal to the child in everyone.

For more information on this book, interested parties may log on to this website:

www.dianatrepkov.com

OUR MISSION *Educate children on personal safety *Increase the awareness about issues relating to missing children * Increase self-confidence in young children*Reduce the statistics of missing children

Endorsements for

I'm Daisy the Safety Chihuahua

Diana Trepkov is a nice person who works with the police, and she draws pictures of missing kids, and the police tries to find them. Detectives help find them too. My name is Derek, and I was the first person to read this book (other than Diana). I liked it, and I think you will like it too! This book will help you a lot if you read it. It will help you to stay safe. It was like Daisy was talking to me. I can read it all the time and lend it to my friends. My wish is that kids should listen to Daisy or to their inside voice to keep them safe and to live a long life.

I remember a time I was going to climb a tree, and I knew I shouldn't have, and I fell and sprained my ankle. I had an inside feeling that I shouldn't, but I ignored it.   **—Derek, age 9**

After reading Diana's (my mom) book, *Daisy, the Safety Chihuahua*, I thought that it is absolutely brilliant to write a fun and safe book about safety for all children. Children need these tips for life to keep safe. This book has smart basic tips for real-life situations. This book is not only for children; it could be for teens as well because a lot of teenagers don't follow through with these tips. They need to be reminded how to keep safe, in my opinion.

Altogether, my mom Diana has done a terrific job writing this book.   **—Nick, age 14**

It was a good book. Diana is smart to teach kids about safety, and another thing that is great about this book is that kids should know not to bully other kids. Overall, it's a great book!   **—Cameron, age 13**

Beautifully written, easy to read fonts, sweetly illustrated and photographed with inspiration and encouragement.

—Grandmother Pauline, age 70

🌷 Author's Note 🌷

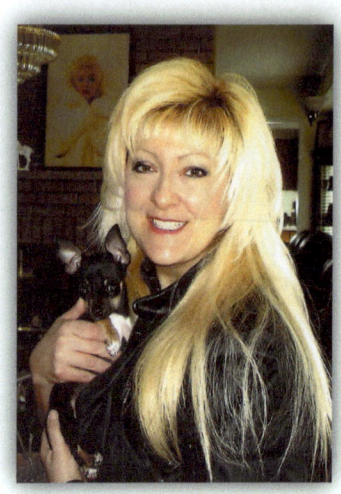

My name is Diana Trepkov.
I have always loved and adored children and animals.
When I was young, I wanted to become a veterinarian
so I could help animals. I never became a veterinarian,
but I did become a forensic artist who helps find
missing people. As long as I am serving others, I feel
like I have chosen the right career as it does not feel
like work to me but something I love and enjoy doing.

Daisy is my puppy dog. She makes me very happy
maybe because she is so innocent, loyal, smart, and
energetic. If I am sad, she is always there to lick my
face, play with me, and cheer me up. She is also a
great watchdog!

My wish for you by reading this book, *I'm Daisy the Safety Chihuahua*, is to find
strength in persevering with any hardship that comes your way. Never, never give
up on your dreams as they are just around the corner! I hope you will adore this
book not only because it's a safety children's book, but because it appeals to the
child in all of us.
You can simply pick this book off your bookshelf, read it, and find yourself being
reminded of all the important safety rules! I would also recommend all mothers to
read this book to their child as it's something they'll remember and cherish when
they grow old. Colorful photographs, detailed illustrations, important safety tips,
and fun activities are all wrapped up in one small package here.

I feel that children of all ages will treasure this book of inspiration, safety rules, and
assurance through their journey in life. Talk to your child frankly and lovingly
about the issues this book raises. Children should always listen to their inner
voice—it is there for a reason and that is to guide them through life. If they pay
attention to their instincts and follow their gut feelings, they will have a greater
chance in living a safe, and joyful life**.**

Everything in life has a purpose, and *if* this book can help save one child from
making an unsafe decision, then this book has fulfilled my goal!

 Much love,
Diana Trepkov and Daisy 🌷

All you need is love.

—John Lennon and Paul McCartney

Dedication

To my dear children, Katrina and Nicholas, I love you both so very much.
Thank you for all the joy you have brought into my life.
To my dear Ava, your smiling face brightens up any room. I love you dearly.
To my dear Anthony, the soccer star, I love you dearly.
May you always stay safe.

I wish for you four to follow your hearts in your lifetime
and believe that anything and everything is possible.
Never give up on your dreams.
They are just around the corner waiting for you.

Thank you, Mother Teresa, for showing the world so much love.
Let us not forget about the missing and abducted children in our world who need
to be found safe and brought home to their families.
To all the victims who cannot speak for themselves,
you are forever in my heart.

This book would not be possible without my loyal friend,
who was there for me every morning as I woke up and wrote this book.
Always happy to see me, sitting by my side, looking up at me with those big loving eyes,
my special little friend, Daisy, the Chihuahua.

Diana P. Trepkov

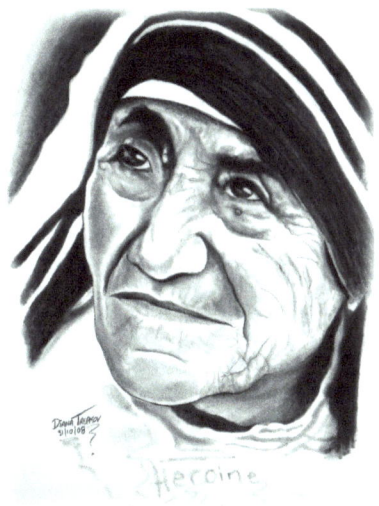

Illustrated by Diana P. Trepkov

Intense love does not measure, it just gives.

—Mother Teresa

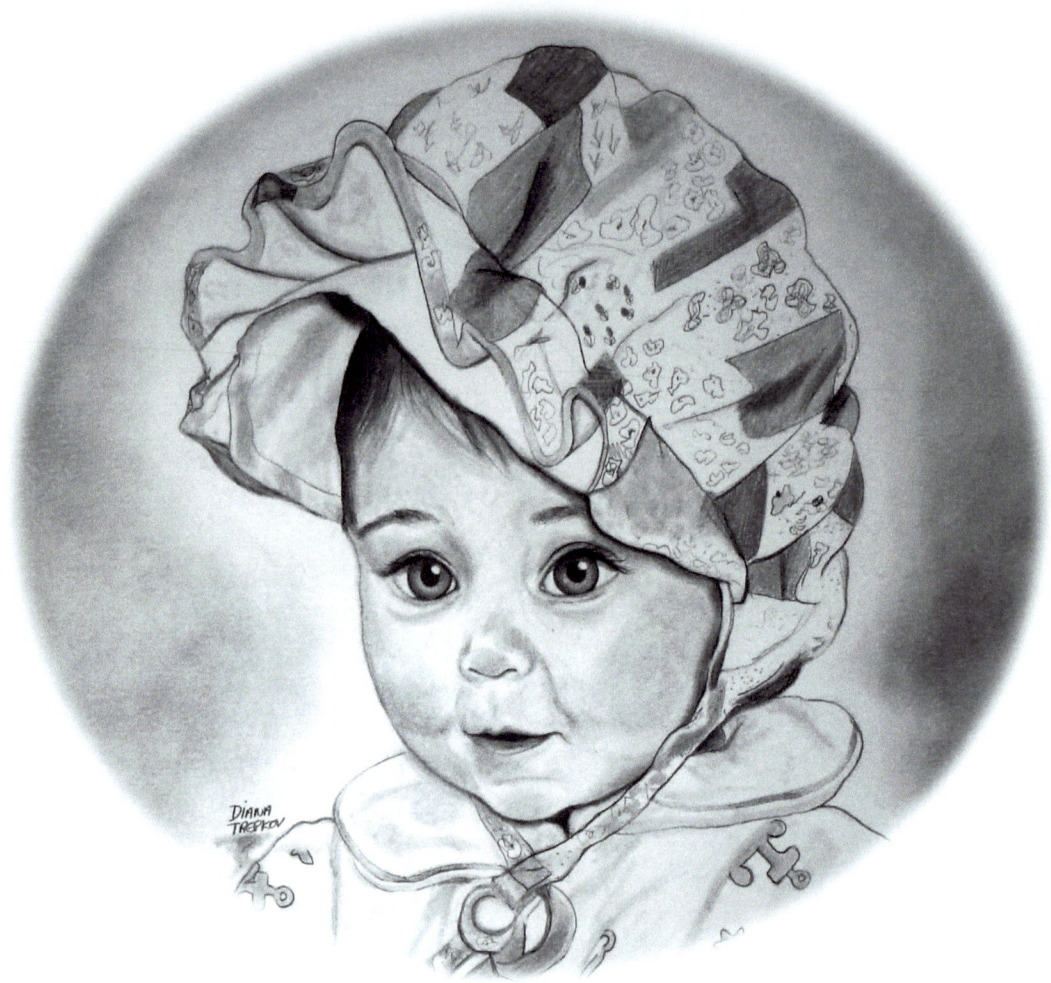

Illustrated by Diana P. Trepkov

Katrina

The meaning of the beautiful name *Katrina* is "blessed, pure, holy."

While we try to teach our children all about life, our children teach us what life is all about.

—Angela Schwindt

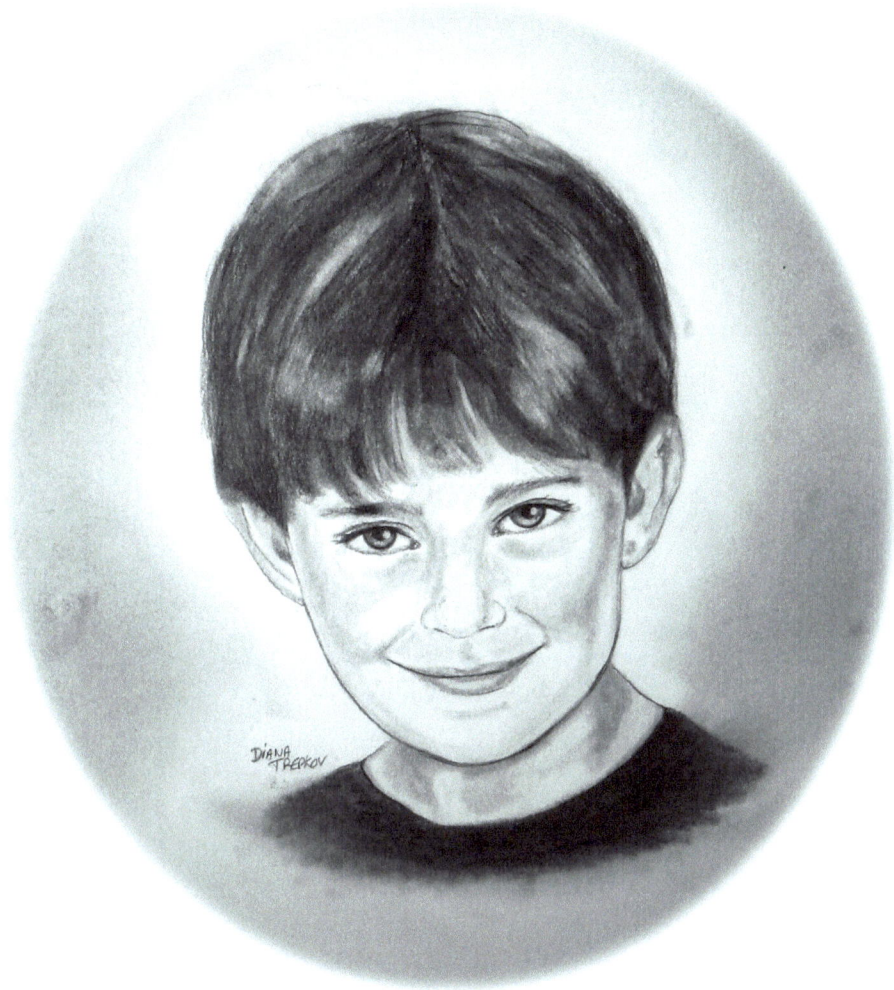

Illustrated by Diana P. Trepkov

Nicholas

The meaning of the handsome name *Nicholas* is "victory of the people."

To the world you may be one person, but to one person you may be the world.

—Brandi Snyder

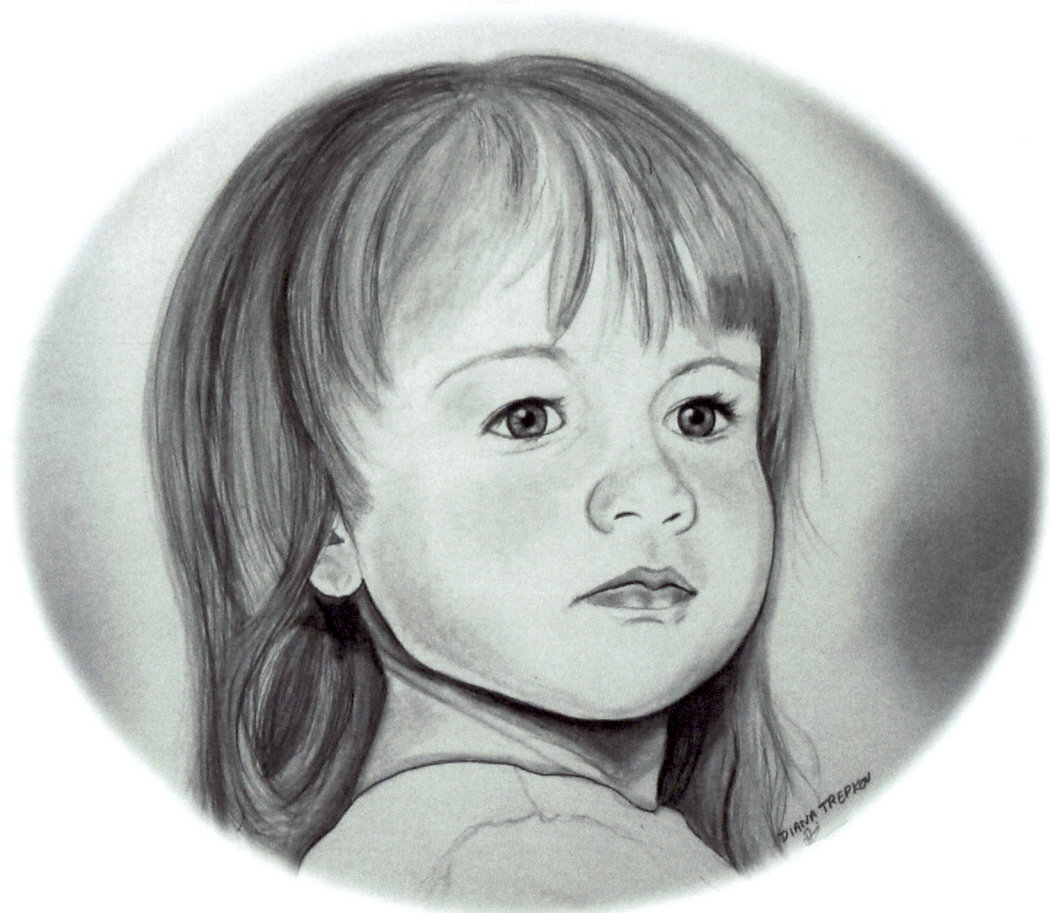

Illustrated by Diana P. Trepkov

Ava

The meaning of the beautiful name *Ava* is "breath of life."

Being deeply loved by someone gives you strength,
while loving someone deeply gives you courage.

—Lao Tzu

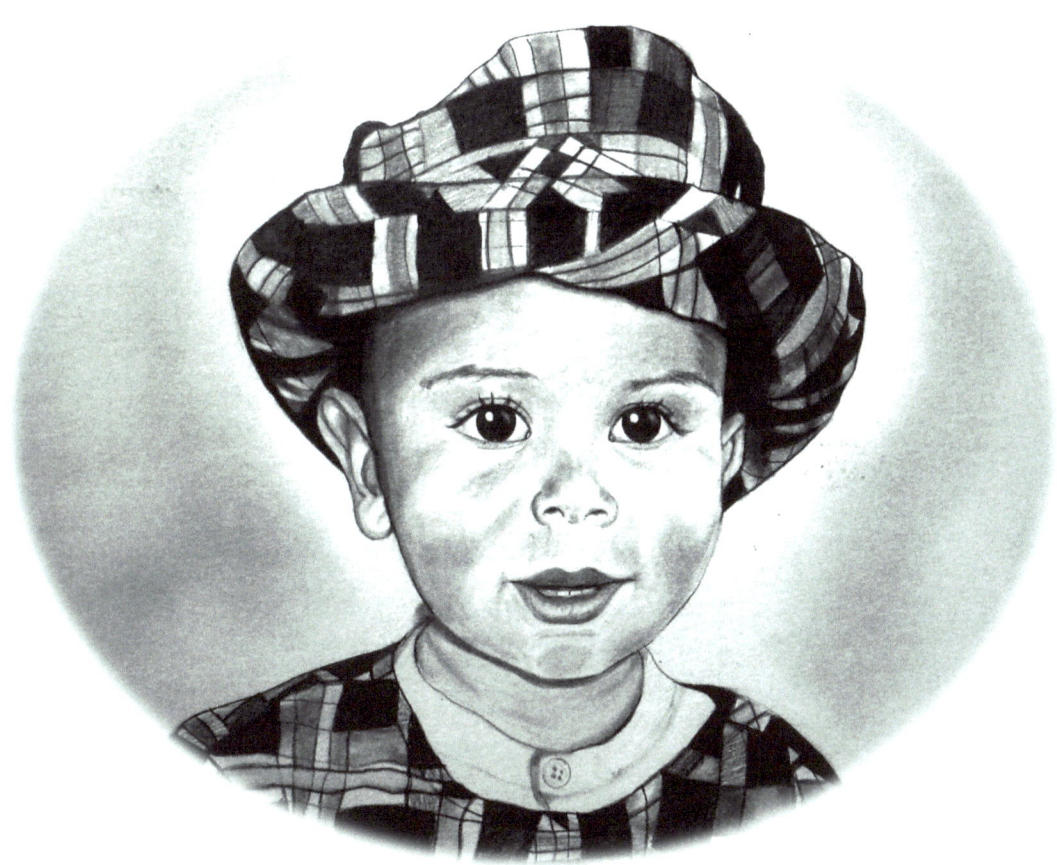

Illustrated by Diana P. Trepkov

Anthony

The meaning of the handsome name *Anthony* is
"a priceless, flourishing flower."

*We are what we repeatedly do. Excellence, therefore,
is not an act but a habit.*

—Aristotle

Preface

Inspired in *St. Paul's Chapel, New York—*
known as the little chapel that withstood/ 911

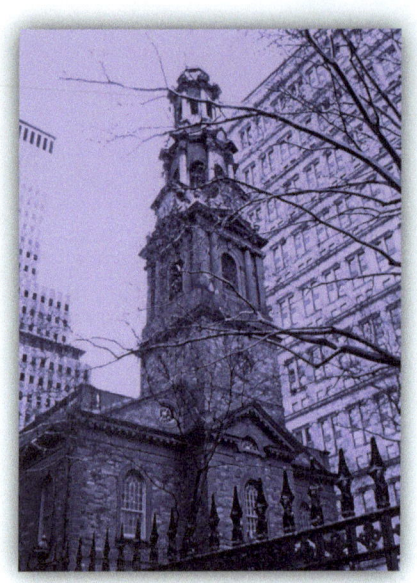

I created, illustrated, photographed, painted, designed, and wrote this book to help show you, the reader, what *forensic art* means to me and how I envision the world through my eyes.

Every parent has a special dream for their children. My dream is to help keep all the children safe in the world.

I was recently in New York City, visiting one of the most beautiful, colorful, multicultural places in the world. Where there is beauty, there is so much more deep within—the sadness of 9/11. Standing next to Ground Zero and walking into the special chapel across the street, I felt my life was just about to change. As I stood in St. Paul's Chapel on April 25, 2011, I experienced many different emotions. I could feel the sadness resulting from the September 11 attack, almost hearing the screams, feeling and visualizing a rush of people in a panic running all over. I felt very sad.

Then suddenly, I started to feel this "special" feeling, like my inner voice was sending me a message, and that was to write this book to help protect the innocent children.

The inspiration I had experienced was unbelievable, overwhelming, and very strong!

St. Paul's Chapel is a very special place; not only did the US president George Washington pray there, it was also the haven for approximately fourteen thousand volunteers offering assistance in the recovery effort of so many people of 9/11. This special chapel was a place of refuge, where food, medical services, rest, and support were provided to the hundreds of rescue workers.

St. Paul's Church is also known as the "little chapel that stood" because it survived the September 11, 2001, attack when the World Trade Center buildings literally collapsed just across the street.

As I stood in St. Paul's Chapel, a very powerful inspirational feeling went through my body. Was someone sending me a message? It was like someone held my hand and brought me to the back of the church; I sincerely felt like I was guided. Then all of a sudden, a million ideas stormed through my head. I couldn't believe this amazing feeling of hope for the future and for the children. It was a miracle!

I thought to myself, *I should write a book with a lot of colorful pictures to represent HOPE and HAPPINESS. I can help protect children with important safety tips.*

It is a wish I have deep within myself to protect as many children as possible and to help ease the pain that I have witnessed in so many families' eyes of missing loved ones. This is written from my heart and through my eyes, the eyes of a forensic artist.

Sometimes we trust the wrong people in life and we believe all people have good intentions, but that is not always the case. Let's educate the children so they can educate their friends, and it will have a life-lasting effect—the ripple effect. I want children to feel safe, happy, secure, and not scared or unsure.

The statistics are too high with so many missing people in the world. Bad guys will be bad guys, and they may want to change, but sadly, they cannot. Therefore, we have to continue to teach all children how to play safe, stay out of trouble, and most importantly, listen to their inner voice, that little voice that guides us and sends us messages throughout.

When I age progress a child who has gone missing to their current age, my heart hurts and burns for them. I can't help but start to worry about what the missing child's family must be going through; it is very sad. My wish is simply to keep the children safe.

Look for the simple but important messages in this book. When you have recognized them, pay attention and remember them!

Abraham Lincoln developed the habit to learn from the books he read and the people he met. Let us follow his footsteps as education, knowledge, and wisdom are the key.

If you let it, this book can tell you how to listen and trust the most important person in the world, and that is you.

Now, it is with such pleasure, honor, and importance that I introduce you to my little friend and puppy dog, Daisy, the Safety Chihuahua!

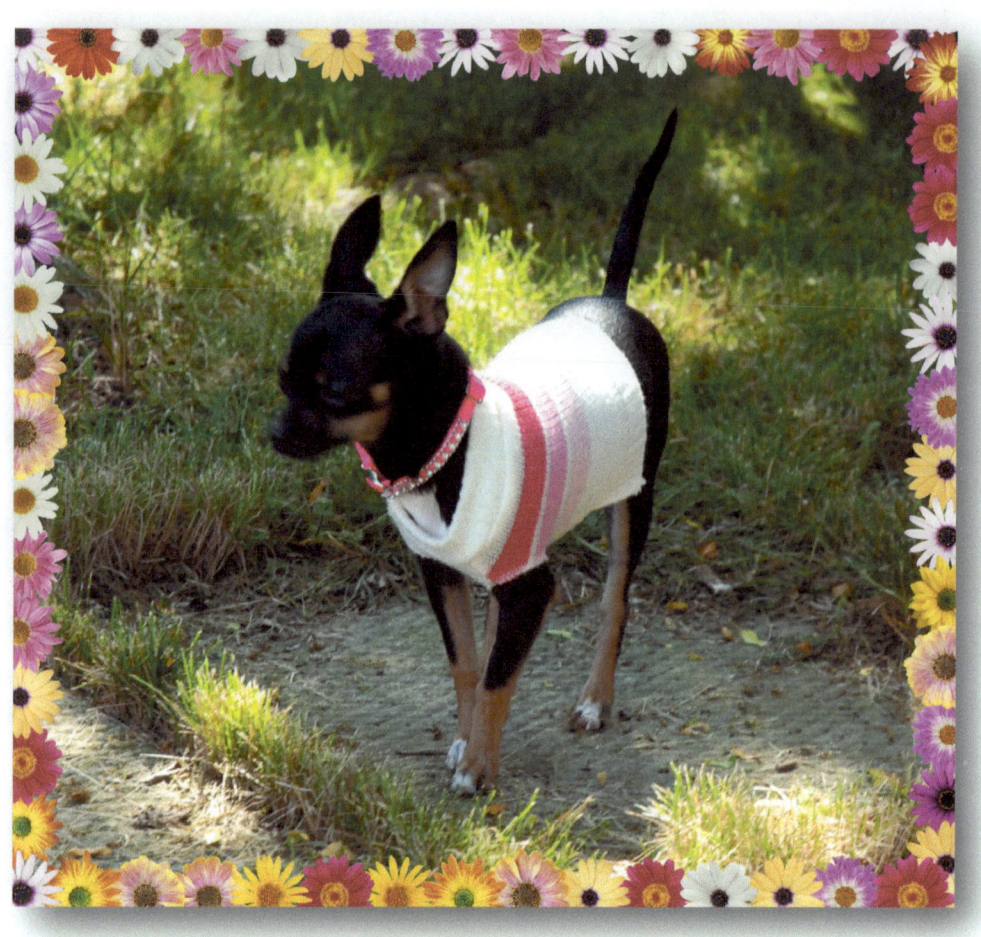

Hello there!
I am so happy you are reading this special book.
My name is Daisy,
and I am a female Chihuahua.
I don't weigh very much at all,
just under six pounds.
Sometimes people don't see me because
of my small size.
I just have to yell, "YIKES!" then they notice me.
I'm the smallest, but I can move quickly
before they step on me!

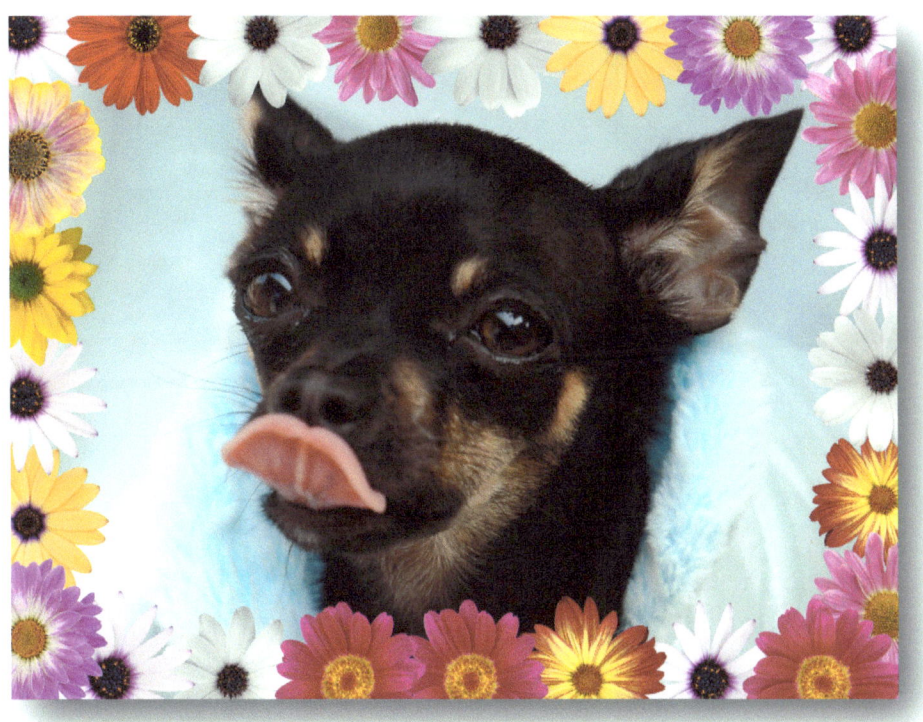

I just finished my dinner; it was yummy!
Good news, now I can tell you what it is like to
have an owner who is a forensic artist.
She helps find missing children with her art!
If a child goes missing, my owner will draw an
age progression of a missing child.
She has taught me so much about staying safe.
I want to share everything I know with you.
It is a true story.
Sometimes I feel sad when I hear
a child is missing.
Do you want to know why?
I feel they should be home with their
moms and dads.
I want to help keep children safe!

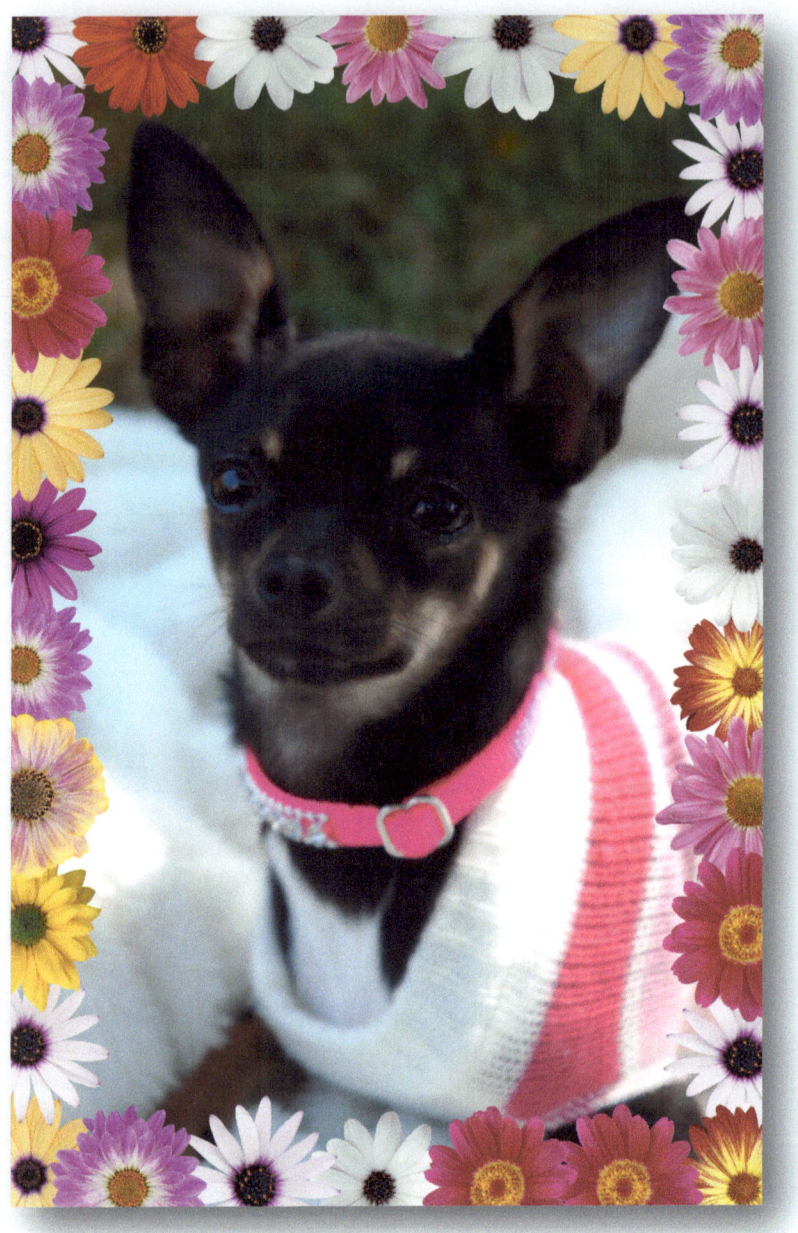

I know you are wondering what it is
I am going to teach you, right?
Well, I have some important safety tips
for you and some good advice.
I have learned a lot by listening with my big ears!

Here are some

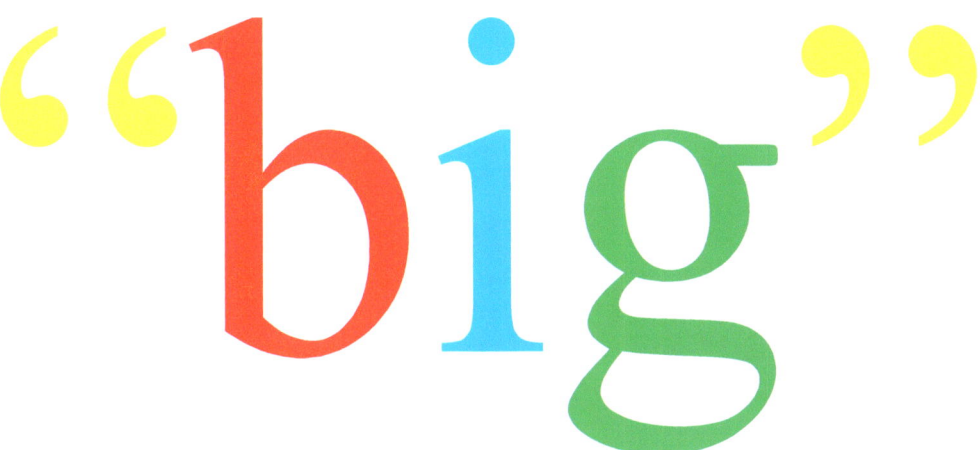

tips that can help you stay safe:

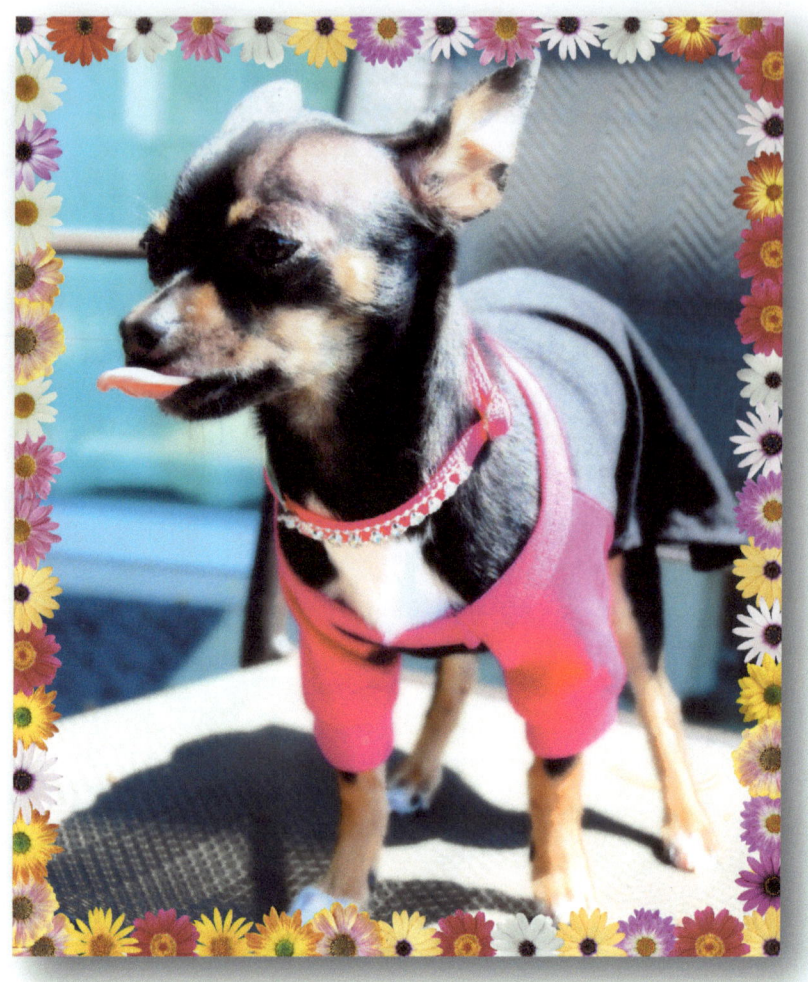

Do not BULLY or MAKE FUN
of other children or people.
Not only is it wrong and very hurtful,
but what goes around comes around.
Remember, everyone wants to be loved. ❤️

If you know someone who is being bullied,
tell your parents or your teacher.
We should all look out for each other as a team.
Try and be a leader and not a follower!

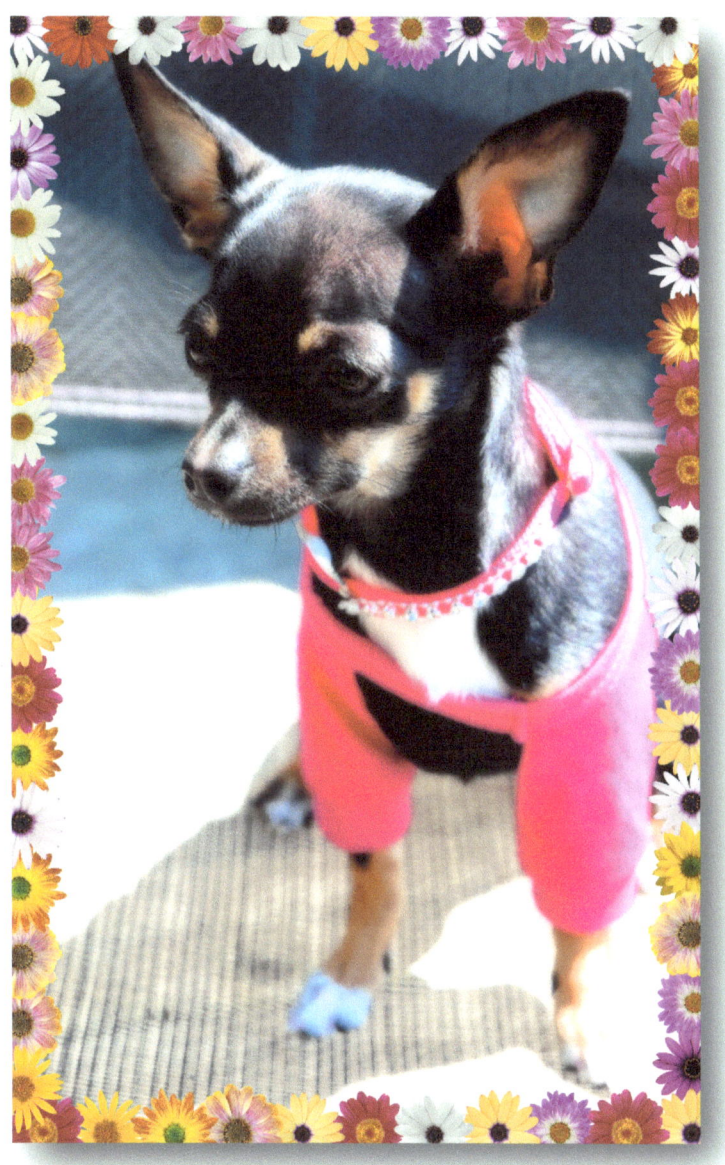

If you are having a bad day and
you are feeling sad,
remember that tomorrow is another day.
Think positive and everything will be fine.
There are always, always, always
great things to be thankful for!
What are you grateful for today? ☀

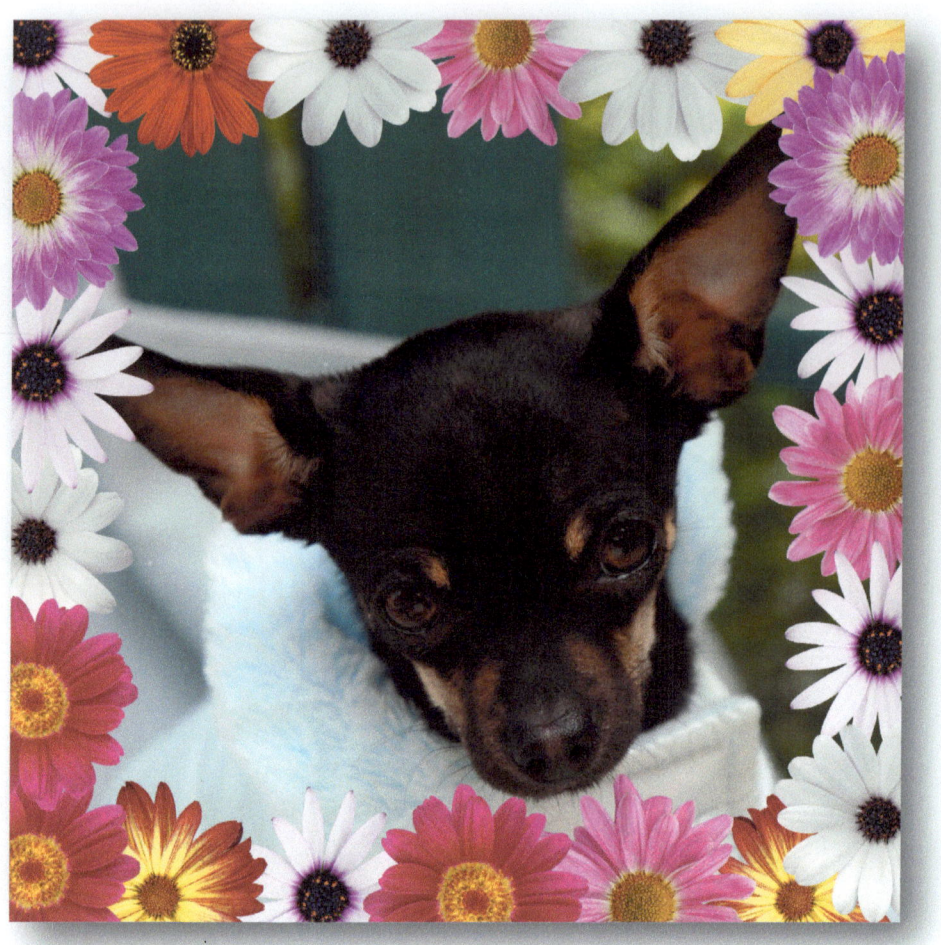

I used to be made fun of because of my BIG ears,
which would make me very sad.
Now I am proud of my big ears because I can
hear better than anyone else!

Appreciate what is different about yourself as we
are all unique and very special in our own way!
Say positive affirmations to yourself
every day . . . something like,
❤️ "I love me—just the way I am!" ❤️

You should have a special secret WORD that only your family knows in case of emergencies. If mommy or daddy can't pick you up, and someone else is going to come pick you up, that person should know your secret family word.
For example, my secret word is "Mexicana."

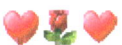

Don't be afraid to tell your parents or a trusted adult if you are worried because something makes you feel uncomfortable or upset.
Communication is very important!

If someone ever tries to grab you and take you away, SCREAM "You are not my MOM" or "You are not my DAD." Yell "FIRE" or just try and make the BIGGEST, LOUDEST noise ever!
I know you can make a BIG noise!

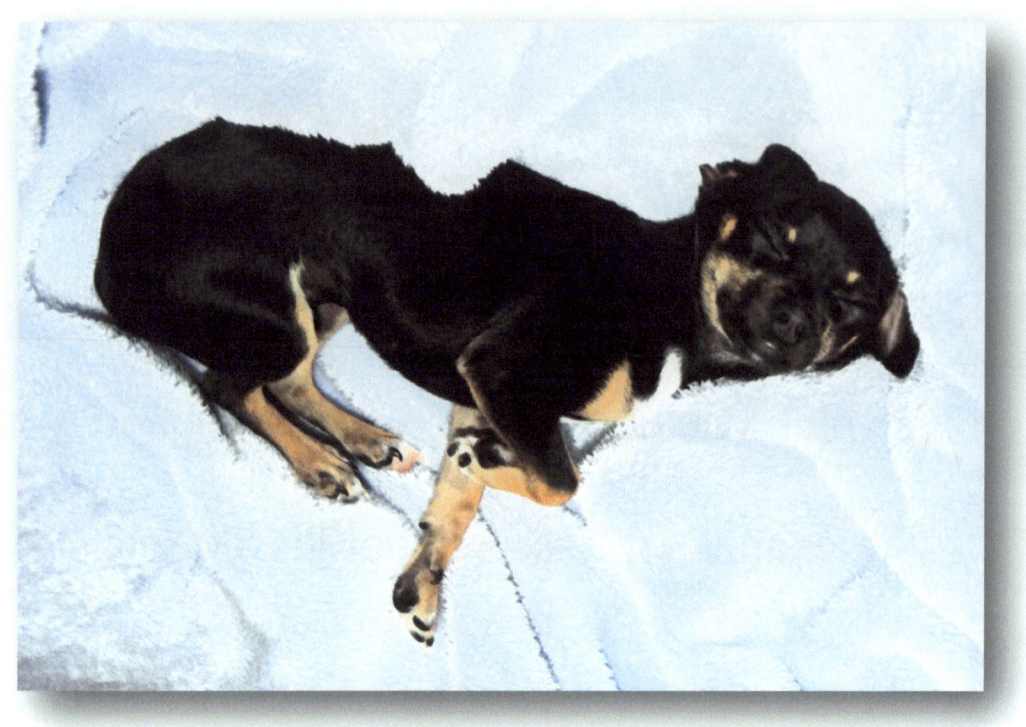

Zzzs . . .

Try to get a good night's sleep.
When you sleep well, you will feel great and
make smart and wise choices!
We all need a lot of sleep so we can grow up to be
healthy and strong.

I always nap when my owner naps!

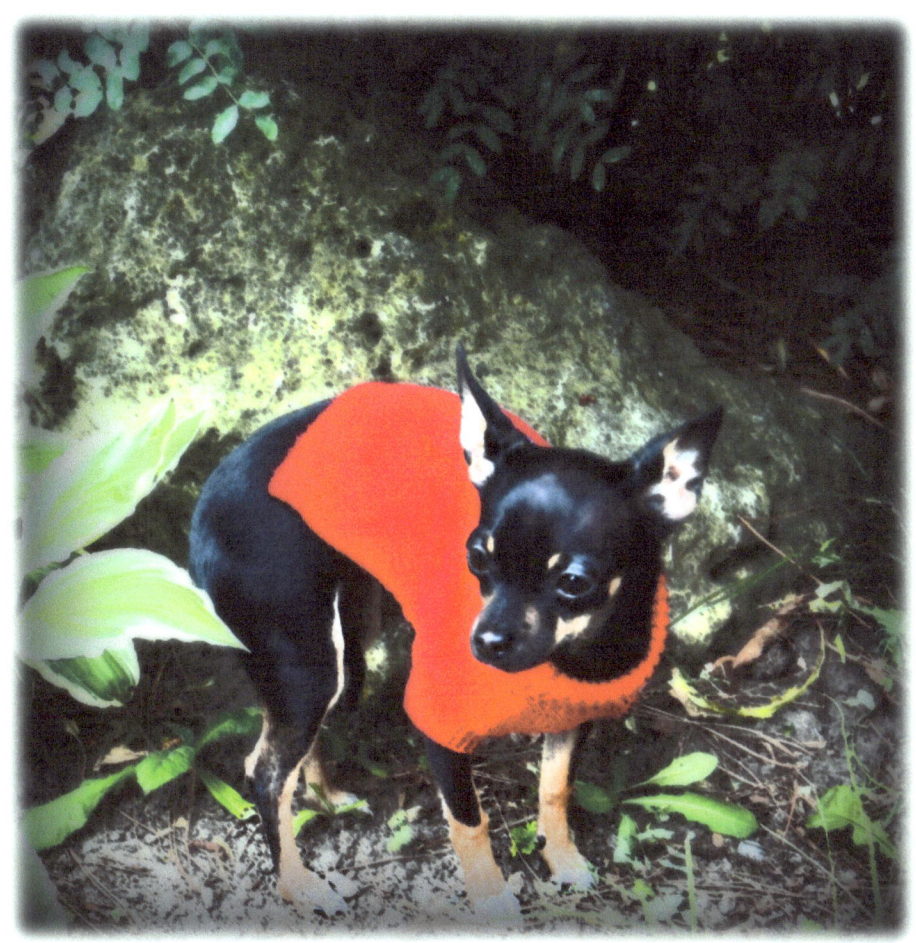

Never walk alone, especially at night.
Always walk with a friend or a parent
or in groups.
Don't approach a car and never
get into a stranger's car.
While crossing the street,
always walk with an adult.
Make sure that you look at both sides
of the road and see that no vehicles are
coming near you.
Make sure your parents know where
you are at all times!

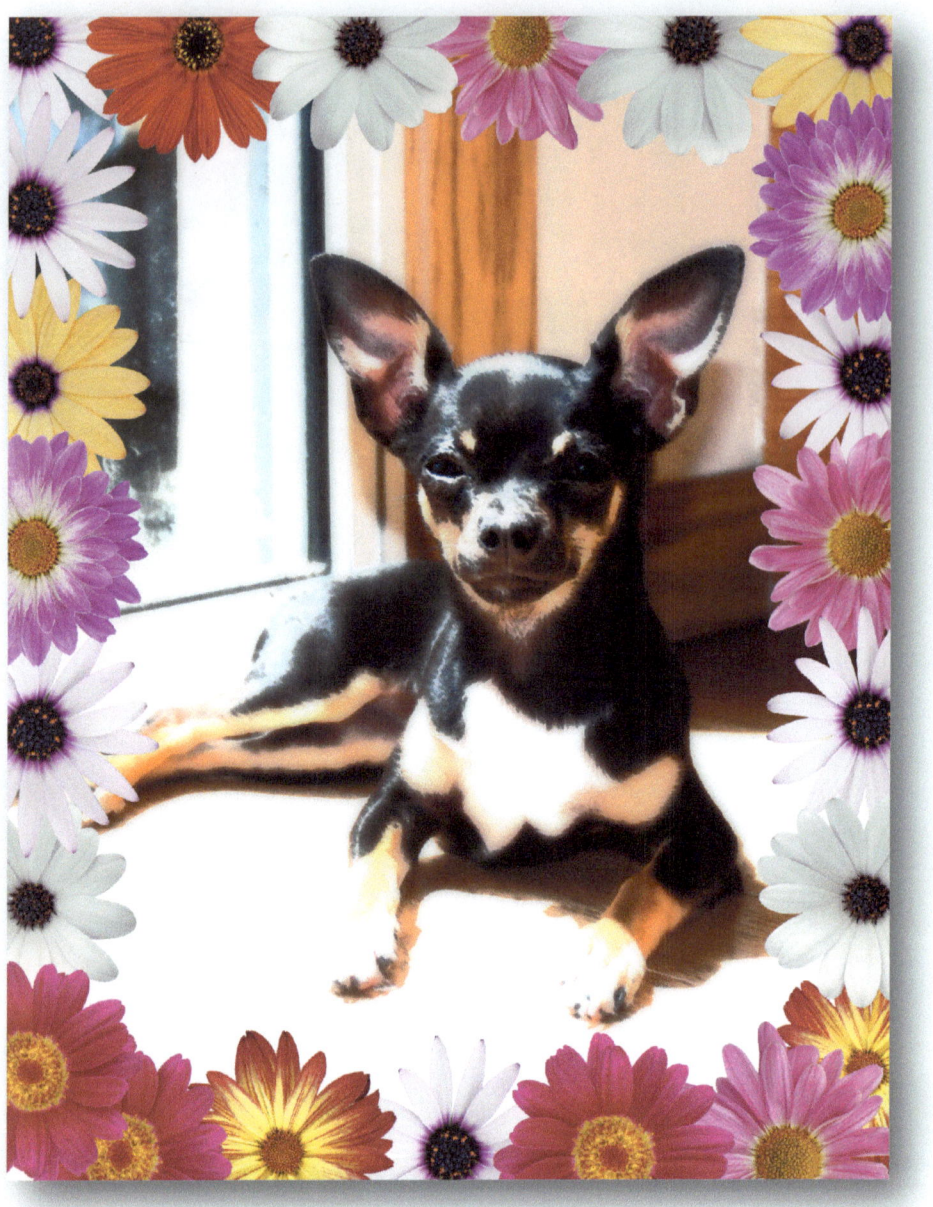

☀️Sunshine brightens my day! ☀️
The sun is our friend, and all of us need some
sunshine to make our day, like it has mine.
It is always better to play out in the sunshine
rather than in the nighttime.

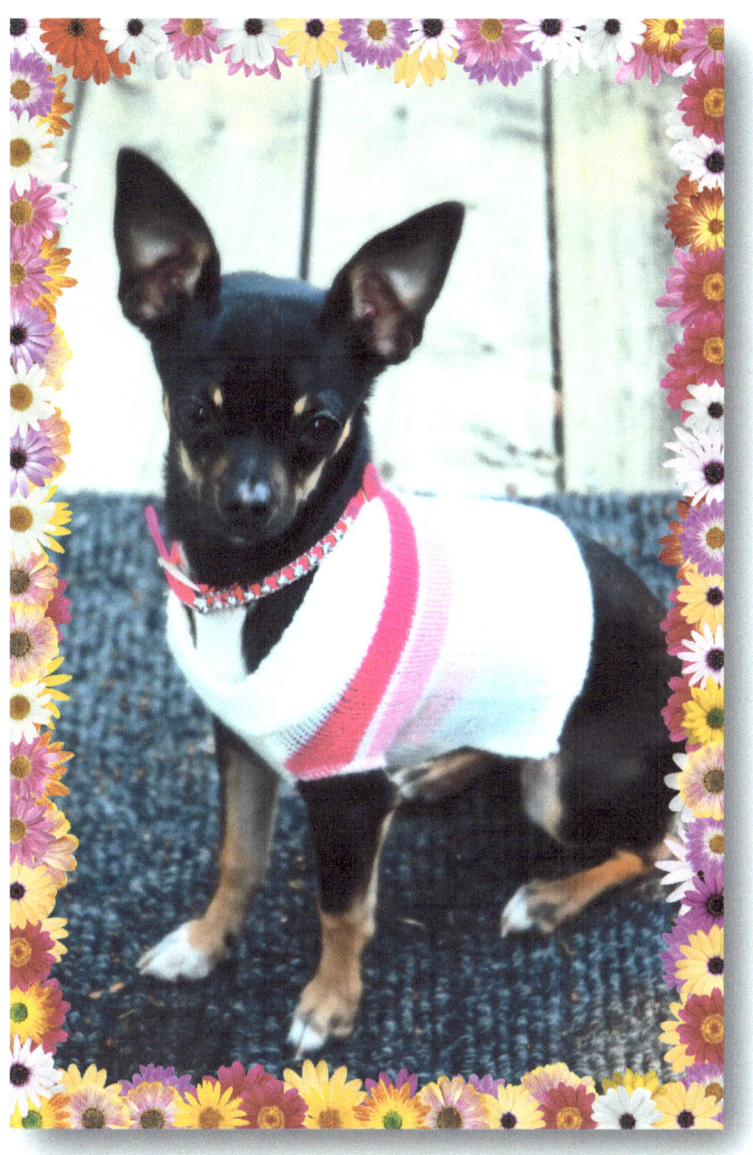

You don't have to always say yes.
If you feel something
is wrong, Just SAY NO!

Don't take candy, food, drinks,
and presents from a stranger.
Always say NO to drugs and alcohol!

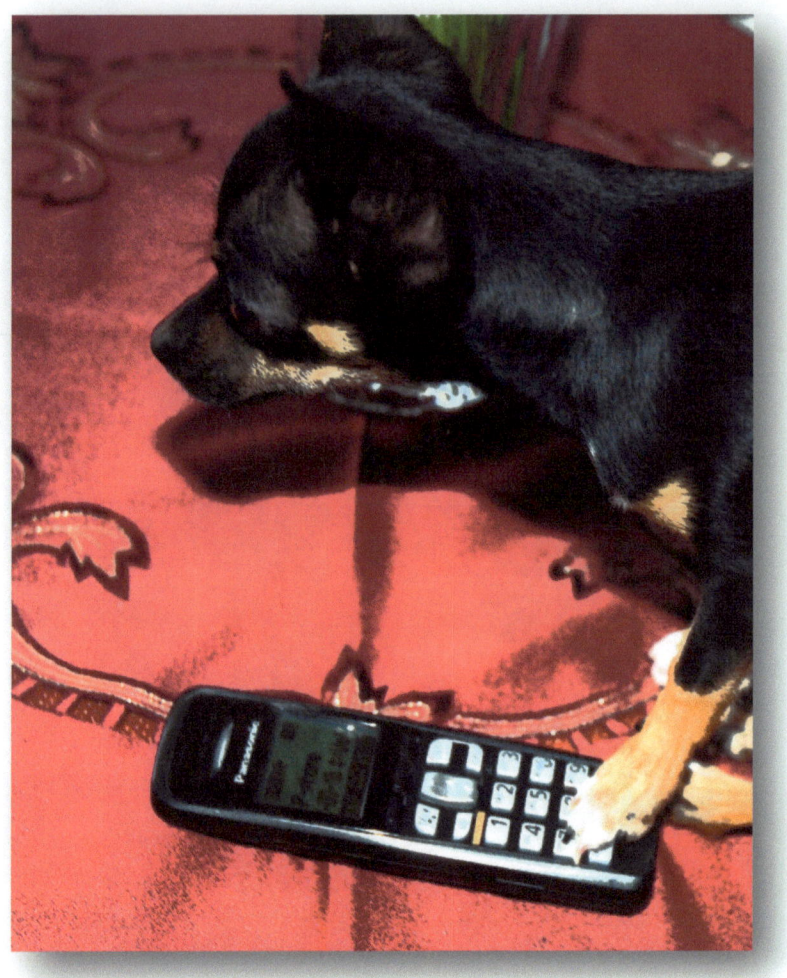

Learn how to dial **911**
for EMERGENCIES at home and at
a public telephone.

If you see a stranger peeking in your window or
walking around your house, call **911**.

To find help—go to a police station, fire station,
or retail shops.

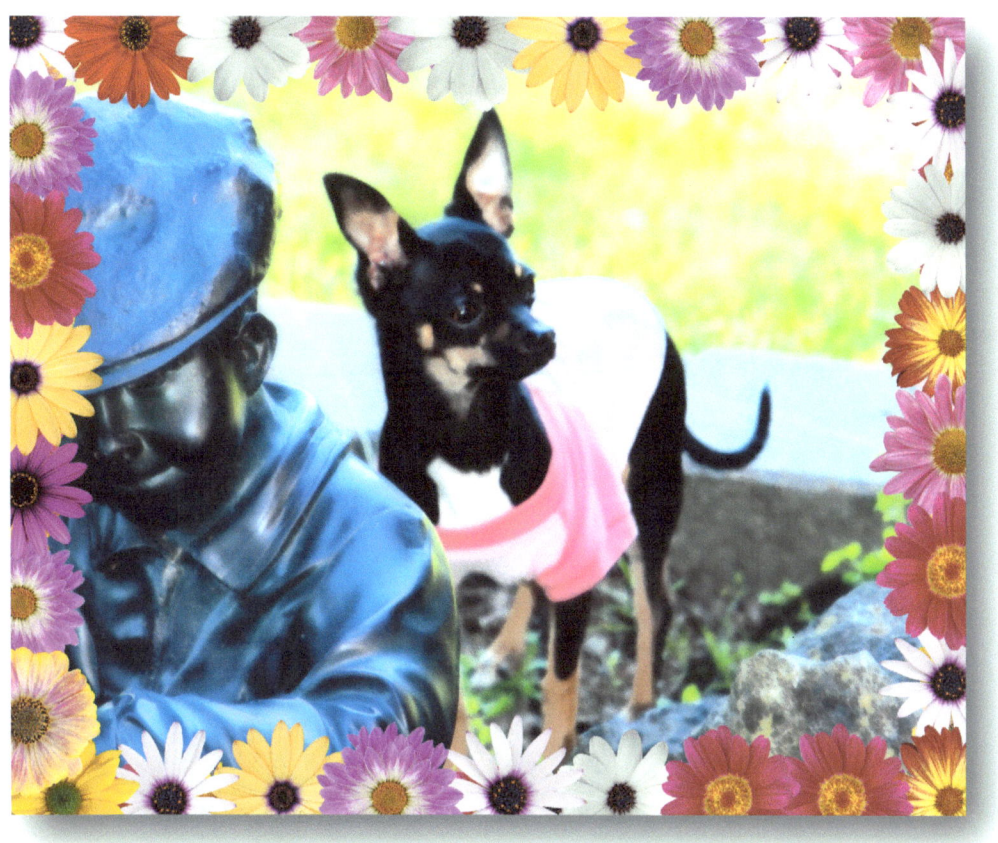

Always be familiar with your surroundings.
Stay away from strangers.
The reason you should never go anywhere with a
stranger is because it is very
dangerous, and I want you to stay safe!
Don't walk alone at night.
Always stay with a group of people.

Information on the computer may not be true;
someone online may pretend to be someone else.
Have your parents by your side
when you are online.
It is better to be safe than sorry!

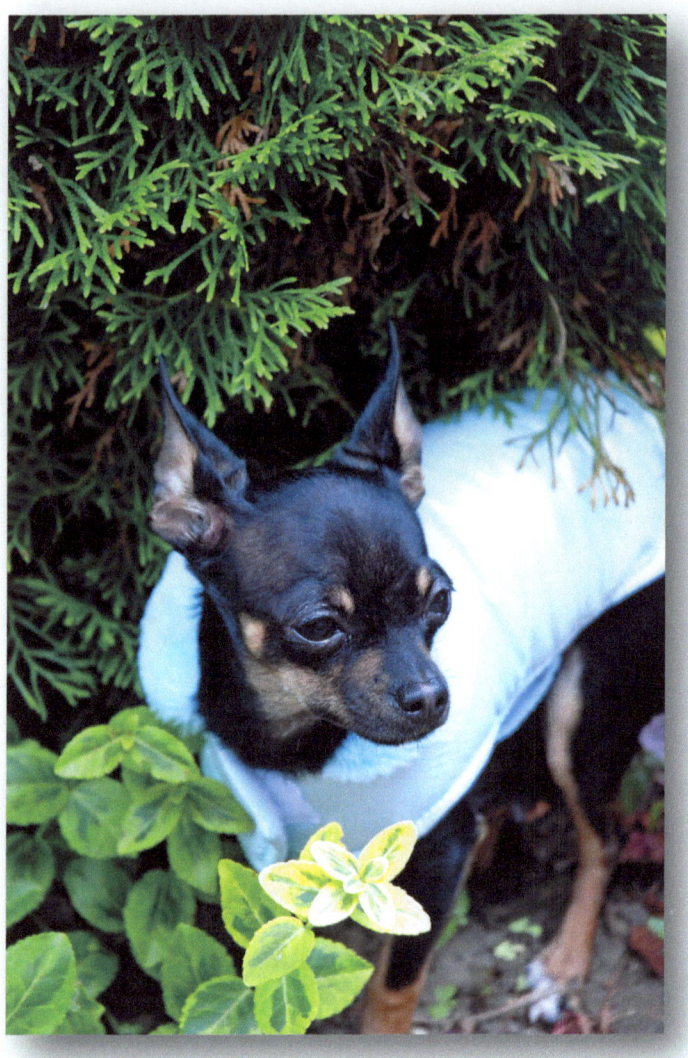

Always trust your feelings and don't ignore them
because that is when we can make bad choices.

We have a special feeling inside
(gut feeling or butterflies in our stomach)
and that is called our instinct or inner voice.
We are so lucky we have this because it is there to
guide us and to protect us through life.

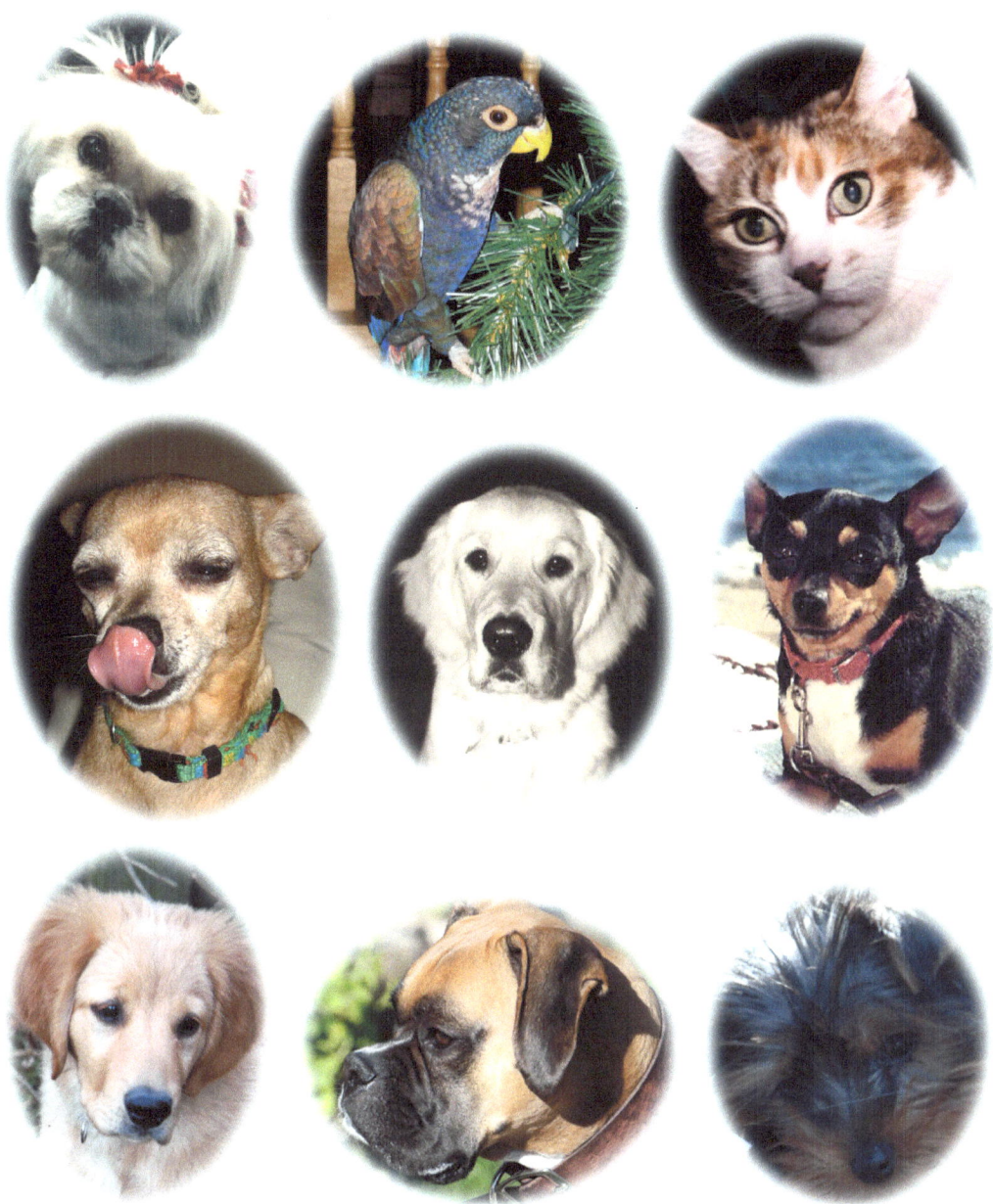

Even though we may look different on the
outside, we are all the same on the inside.
Always be considerate of other people's feelings.
We all hurt the same, we all love the same,
and we all laugh the same.
We are ALL equally important!
🐢🐈🐕🐐🐑🐇

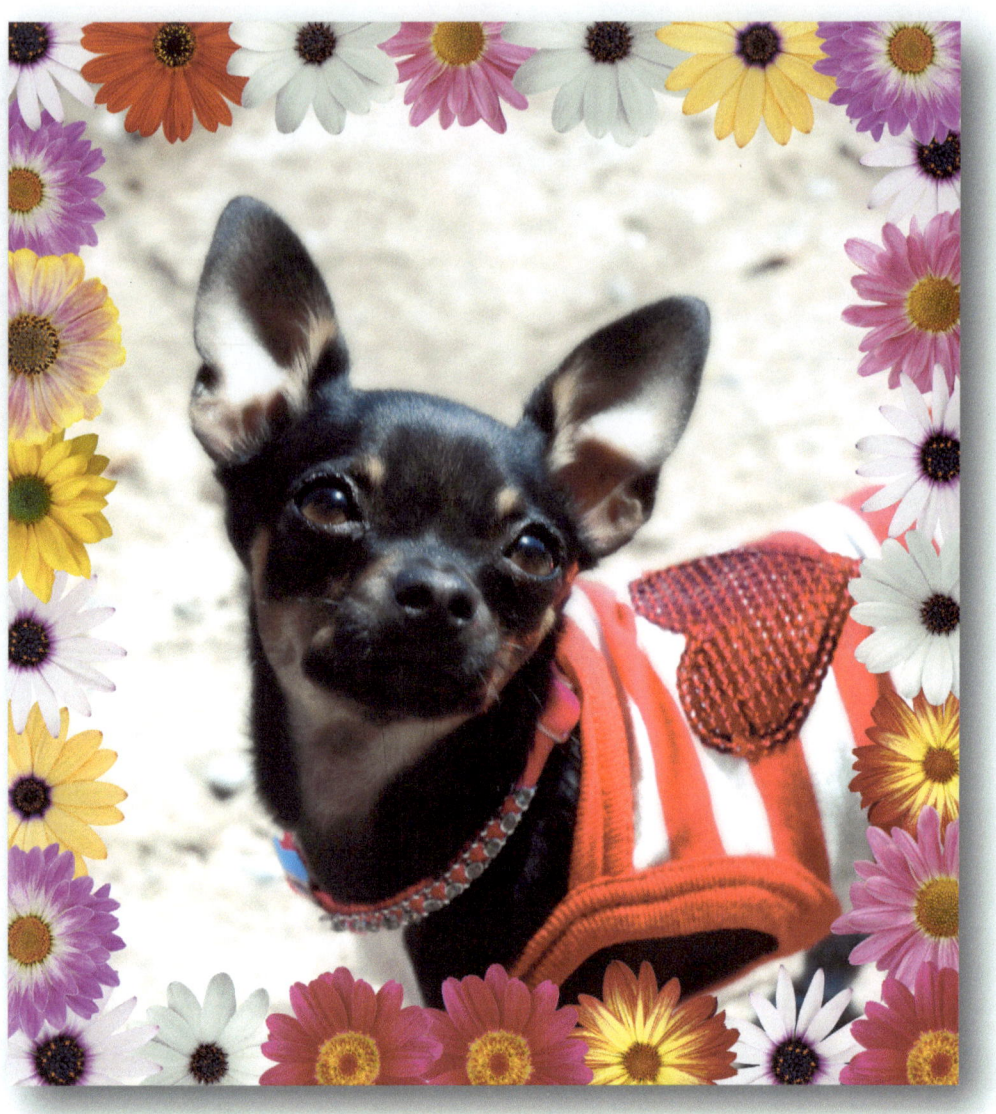

Always speak from your heart.
When we speak from our heart,
we speak the truth. ❤️

Our parents, grandparents, brothers, sisters,
and our teachers are the best listeners.
Let's share our thoughts with them when we are
sad or scared or just need someone to listen.

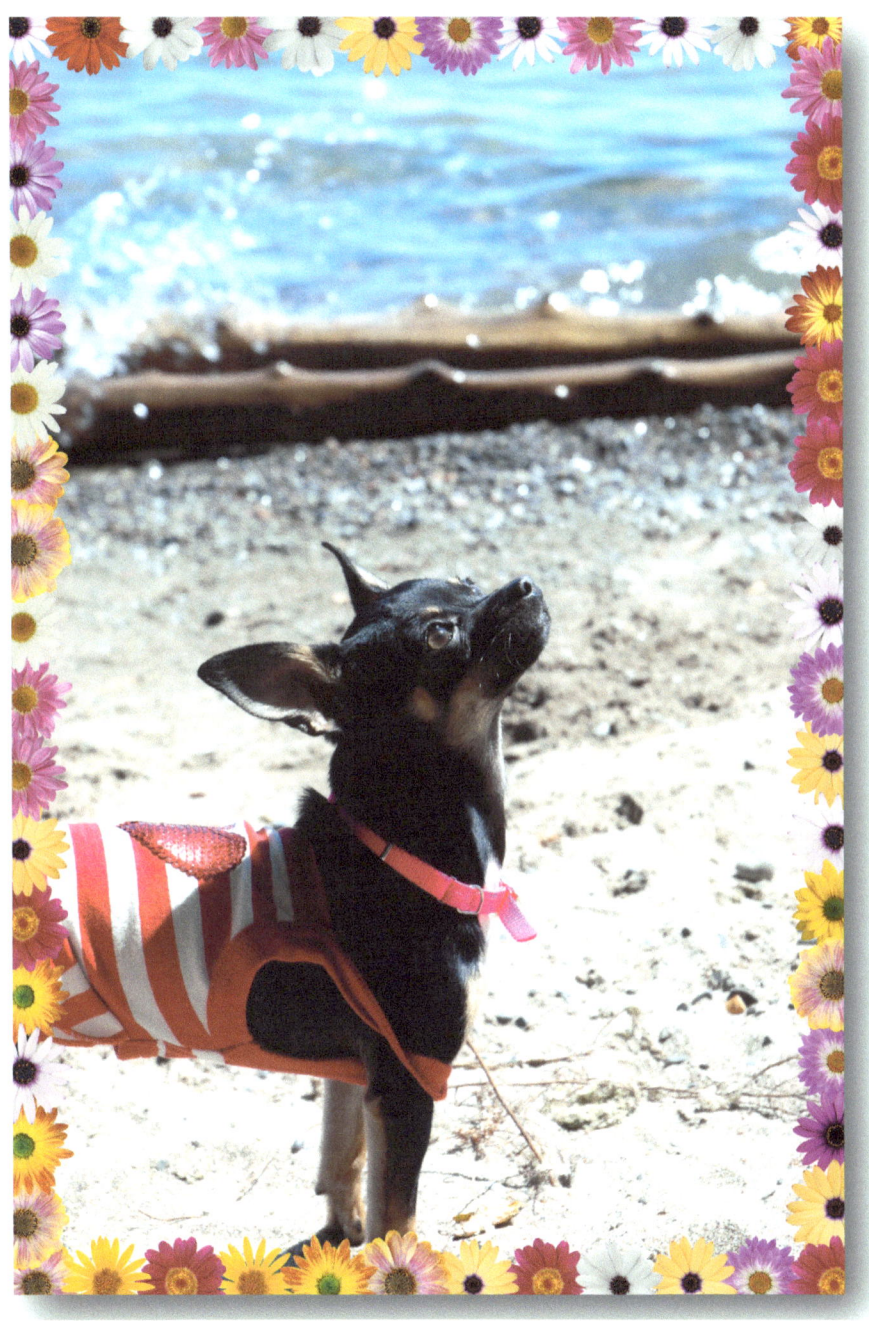

Be open to some good advice.
There are many great leaders and teachers in the
world. Listen, learn, and then apply!
Learning is so much fun!

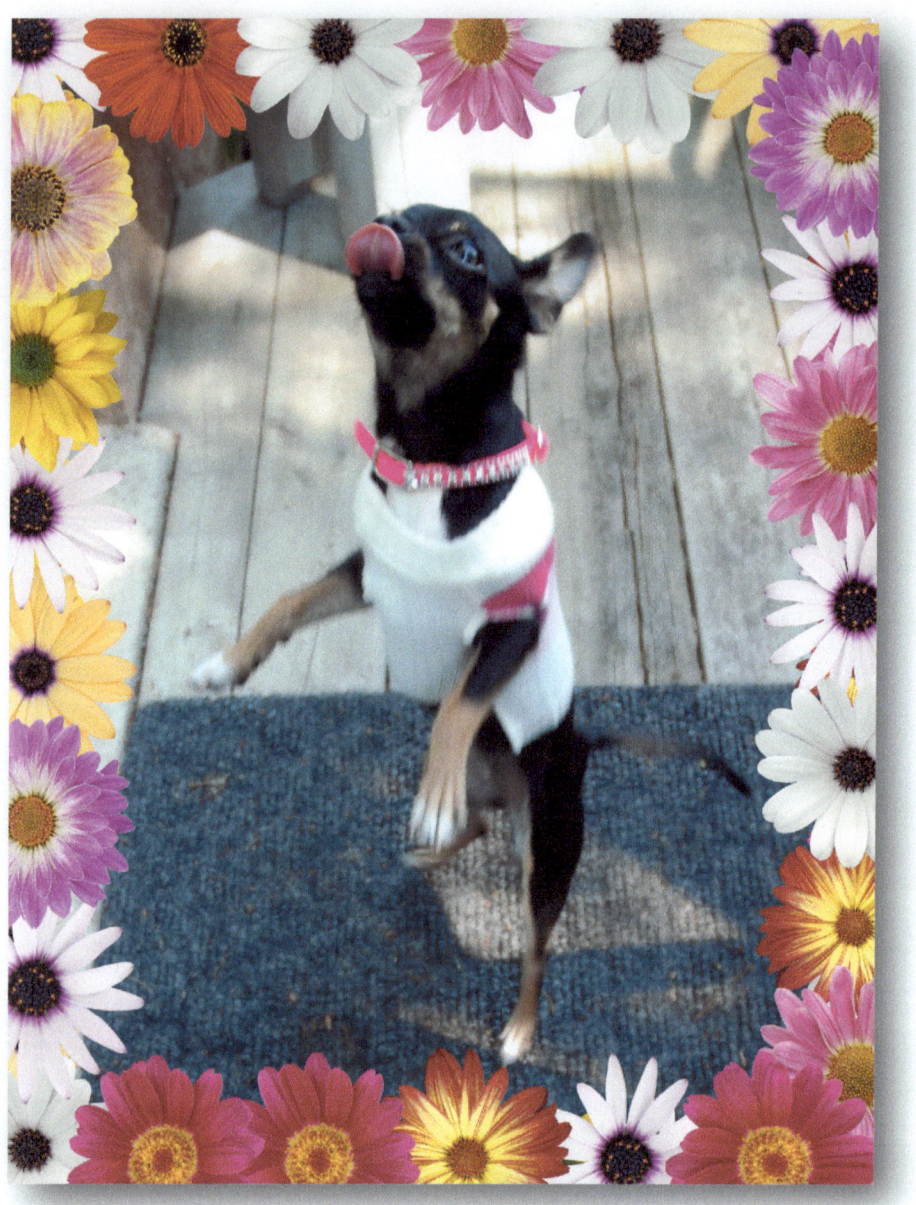

Have fun and dance to some great funky music!
What kind of music do you enjoy listening to?
I love all kinds of music! ♪
I have always loved to dance and imagine that I
am a princess and twirl around!

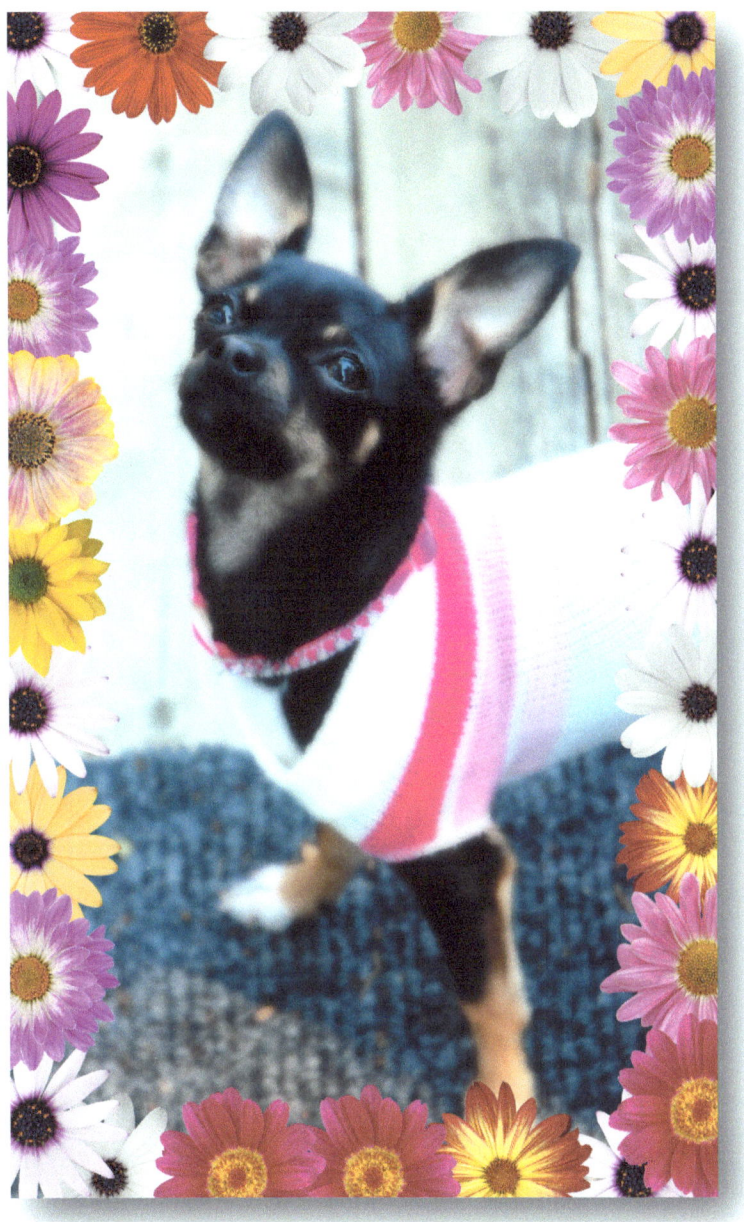

I want to say thank you so much for reading my safety book! I poured my heart and soul into it. This book will give you a lot to think about.

Can you think of ways to play safely?

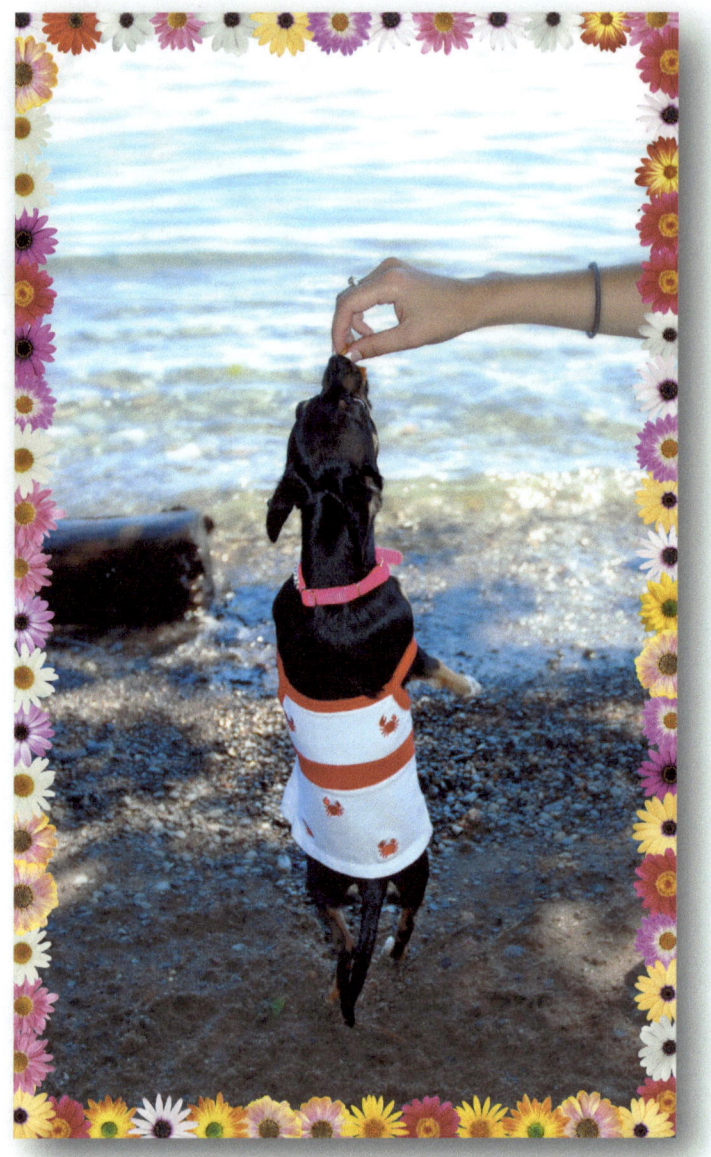

Today is a very special fun day!
I love dancing on the beach and eating yummy food!
I wish you lots of joy today and every day!
I think you should have a party with all your special
friends and share what you have learned about
safety and having fun!
Follow your heart and always BELIEVE in yourself.
Never, never give up on your DREAMS!

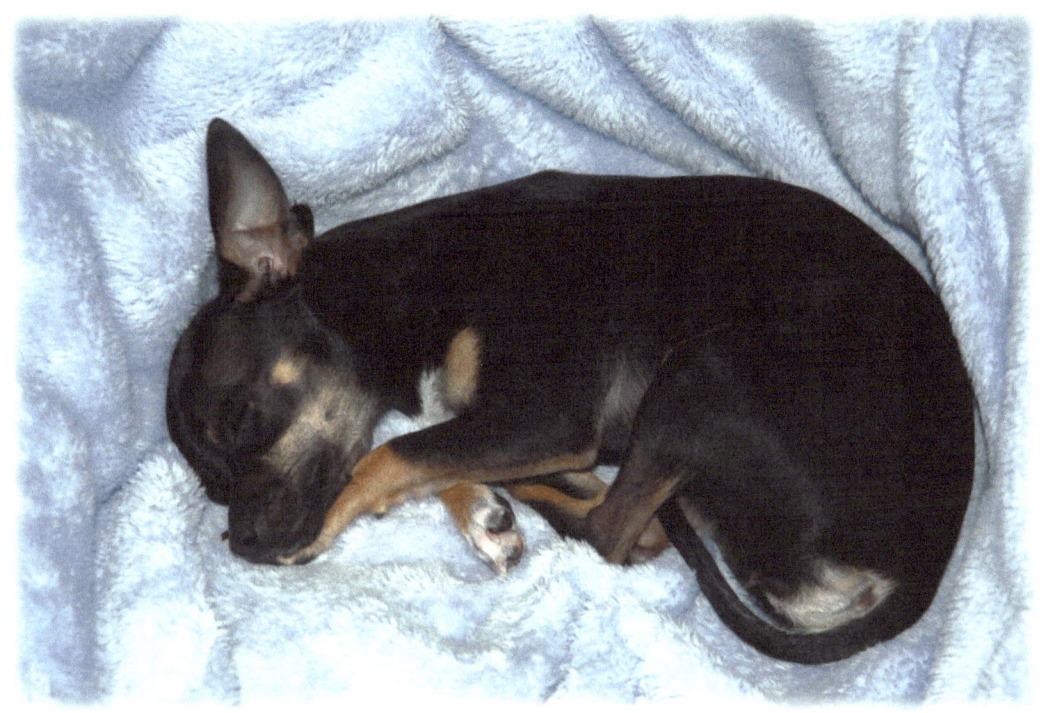

Now it is time for bed . . .
my dream for you is to always stay safe because I
will love you unconditionally and
I will love you forever.

Good night.

Sleep tight . . . zzzs . . . 🌈

The End.

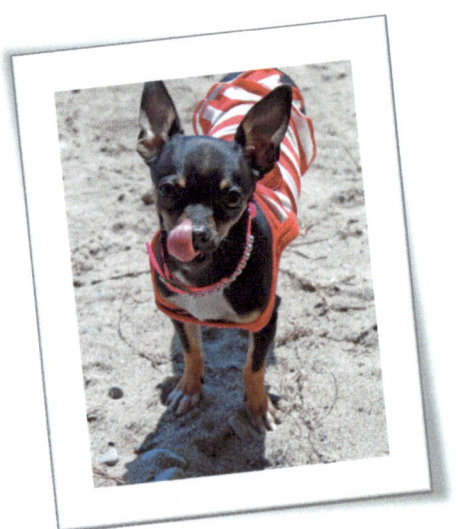

Don't cry because it's over. Smile because it happened.

— Dr. Seuss

NOTES
What did you learn from this book?

1.) _____

2.) _____

3.) _____

NOTES
How can YOU continue to stay safe?

1.) _____

2.) _____

3.) _____

NOTES
How can you help some child feel safe when he or she is scared?

1.)_____

2.)_____

3.)_____

NOTES
SELF-LOVE: List three things that you love about yourself!

1.)_____

2.)_____

3.)_____

NOTES
List three things you love to do that makes you feel joyful when you do them!

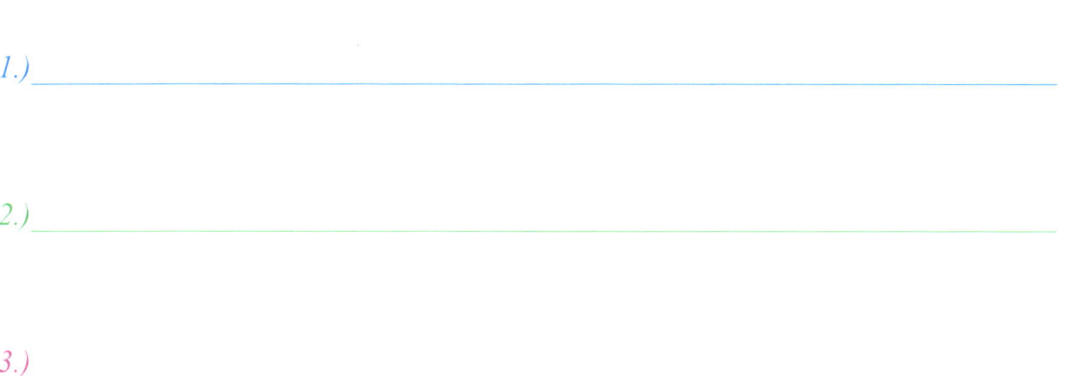

1.)_____

2.)_____

3.)_____

NOTES
The BEST things in life are free!
What are three special surprises you can do today to show someone you care?

1.)_____

2.)_____

3.)_____

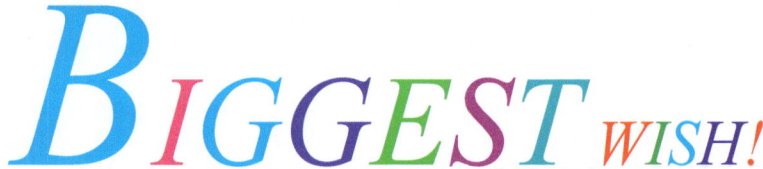

NOW think OF something THAT YOU
really, really, really want.
Now write it down!
⭐⭐⭐

Promise me
you will always remember—

You are braver than you believe,
stronger than you seem,
and smarter than you think.

—Christopher Robin to Pooh

ARTIST
Draw a picture of something you love!

Coloring Page

Be aware of your surroundings.
Not everything is as it appears to be.
Do you want to **Color** this picture?

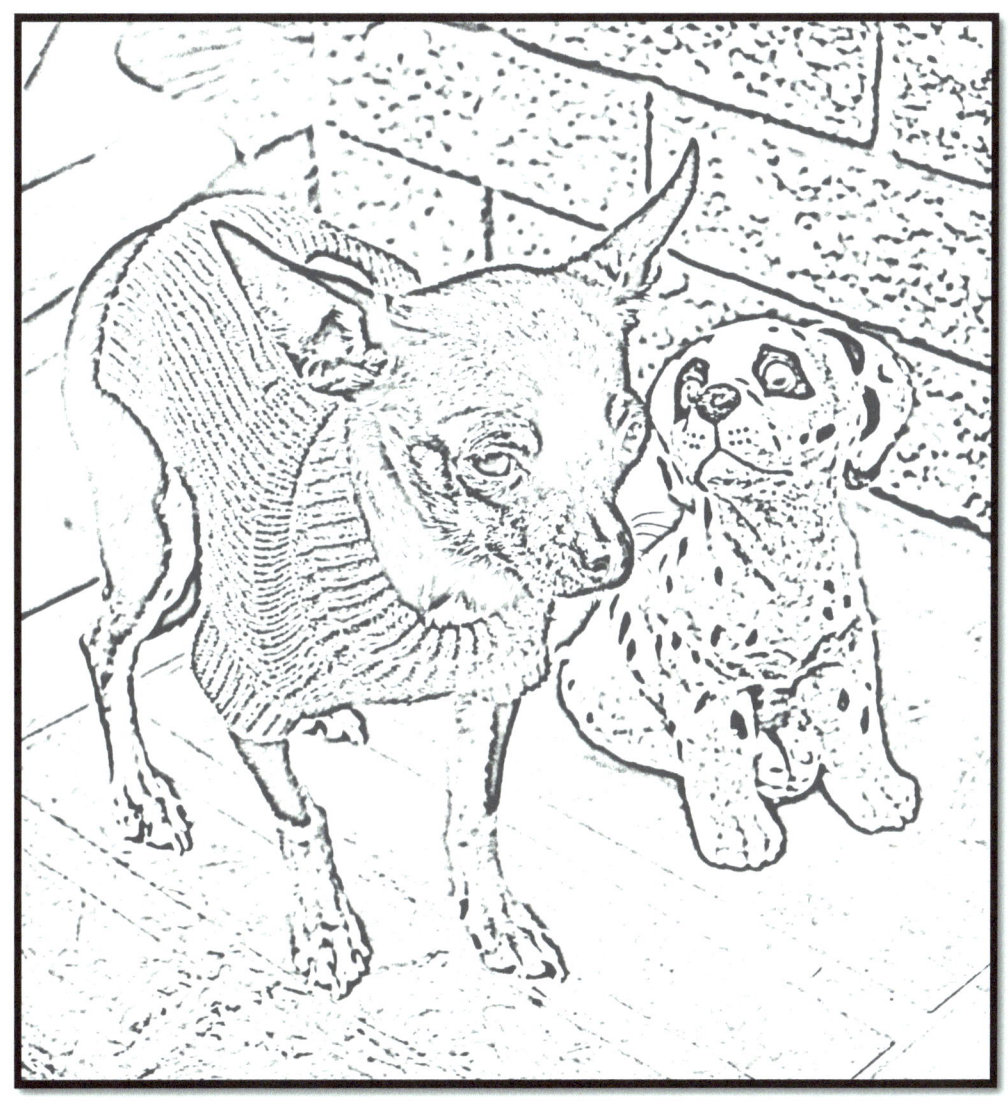

Coloring Page

My owner is a forensic artist, and she is drawing
a missing child's age progression.
Do you want to **Color** this picture?

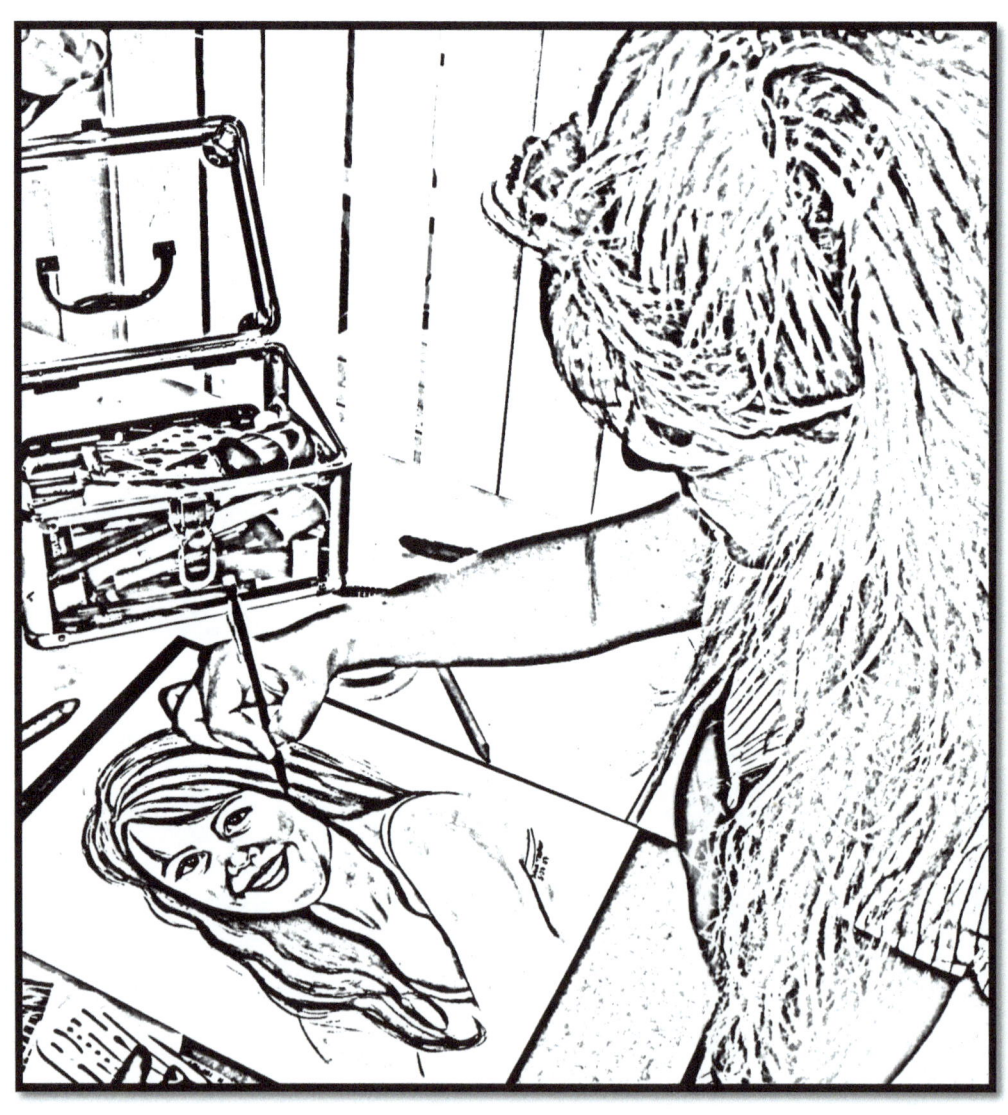

A baby cheetah is one of my favorite animals!

I think you should get a sheet of paper and paint one of your favorite animals. You will do a great job on it!

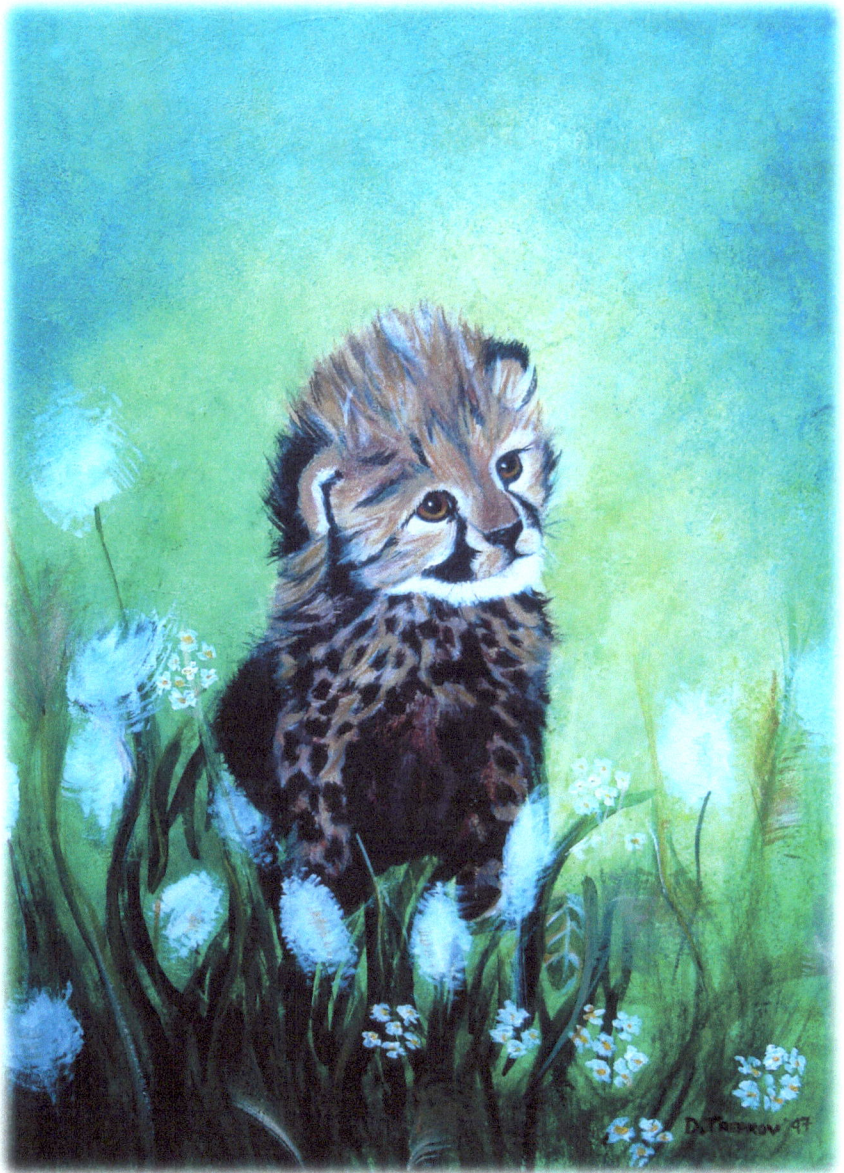

Painted by Diana P. Trepkov

Do you love me because I am beautiful, or am I beautiful because you love me?

—Cinderella

🌷 Special Notes for Teachers and Parents 🌷

~Look at any photo of Daisy, the Chihuahua.
Tell the children how you feel about this puppy.
Now ask the children how they feel about this puppy.
Also, ask the children how they think this puppy feels.
Ask about their special pets or favorite animals and why.

~Ask the children what they are afraid of.
Discuss with the children what these fears are and why.
What do you think can help take these fears away?
Discuss why following safety rules can help keep all children safe.

~Ask the children to tell you the favorite part of this book and to explain why.
Tell them what your favorite part of this book is and explain why.

~Talk about the important lessons of safety in this book.
Ask the children why it is very important to follow their inner voice,
which is also called "intuition."
You could tell them a story about how your intuition saved you
from a bad experience and guided you to safety.

~As a group discussion, ask the children about some other important
safety rules that might have not been
mentioned in this book that they would like to share.

~Ask the children what their names are. Discuss the meaning of their names.

~Ask the children if they can share what they learned on how to stay safe.
Discuss how they can help others to stay safe!

Attention: Parents, Schools, and Businesses
This book is available at quantity discounts with bulk purchase for educational,
business, organizational, or sales promotion use.

E-mail: **dianatrepkov@rogers.com**

Logic will get you from A to B. Imagination will take you everywhere.

—Albert Einstein